Gentle Illustrated Yoga
Handbook for your Back

Illustrated by Simona Molino
Translated by Simona Silva

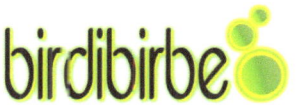

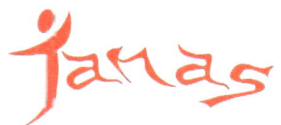

This handbook is for information only and does not supersede any medical or psychological treatment.
The illustrations are also purely informative.
Readers, by deciding to assume the illustrated positions, do so at their own risk and and under their own full responsibility.

Supine Positions

Savasana or Corpse Pose

Jathara Parivritti Asana or Belly Twist Pose

Pavana-mukta-asana or Wind-relieving Pose

Dvi Pada Pitham Asana or Little Bridge Pose

Prone Positions

Adavasana or Reverse Corpse Pose

Naga-Asana or Cobra or Snake Pose

Sitting Positions

Dandasana or Staff Pose

Pascimottanasana or Caterpillar Pose

Standing Positions

Tadasana or Mountain Pose

Kala Asana or Time Pose

Padahastasana or Hand under Foot Pose

Namaskarasana or Prayer Squat Pose

Kneeling Positions

Balasana or Child's Pose

Shashankasana or Hare Pose

Quadrupedal Positions

Bidalasana or Cat Pose

Office Poses

Elongating Pose

Uktanasana or Chair pose

Arm stretching while you are sitting

Advice on how to use the Gentle Illustrated Yoga Handbook for your Back

The spine is the central axis of our body.
It is crossed over by numerous nervous bundles connecting vital organs to the brain and has very many functions, such as sustaining the bone joints, the muscles and the skull, providing the dynamic and static balancing of the body and fastening the rib cage, which is directly linked to the breathing process.

A sedentary life, limited exercise and the gravitational attraction while we are standing often generate rigidity and tension in our back and create psychophysical imbalance and illness.
Through experience and the practice of Asanas, Yoga helps us free our bodies from blocks, rigidity and tensions and allows us to find lost flexibility, elasticity and psychophysical well-being.

The Asana postures presented in this handbook will help you, through constant practice, to gradually regain control of your body and to better understand the importance of your back.

Practice Yoga for your Back at any time during the day and give your body a well-deserved rest as well as silence and lack of external pressures.
Some soft background music will help you with your practice.
Tune in to your body and respect its limitations.
Keep a few cushions close for help in certain Asanas and a blanket in case you feel cold in the ground Asanas, such as Savanasana.
If you decide to practice in the open air, you may find a mat useful and your musical background will be live from nature.
Please pay attention to the "Benefits" and "Warning" sections for each Asana and, if in doubt, consult a professional as not to incur in structural damage or worsening of a condition.

 Enjoy!

Savasana or Corpse Pose

The name Savasana comes from the Sanskrit

शव Corpse आसन Asana

The term 'Shava' means 'Having the Appearance of a dead Human Body' and the term 'Asana' means 'Pose'; the body lies in fact supine on the ground, completely relaxed and still.

This pose is also called 'Mritasana', from 'Mrit', meaning 'Dead' and 'Asana' meaning 'Pose'.

Lie on your back with your legs slightly apart, extend your toes outwards; rest your arms slightly apart from your torso with your palms facing upwards, your fingers must feel soft and relaxed.

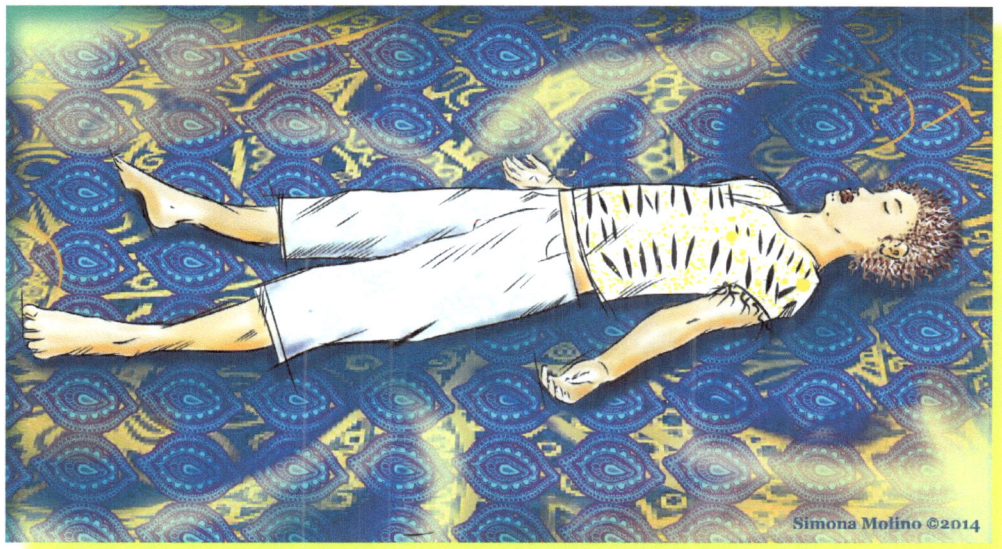

Simona Molino ©2014

Your jaw is relaxed and you tongue rests on your palate.

Close your eyes and breathe normally.

Sense the feelings in your body, starting from your toes to your calves and thighs; now concentrate on your bottom, belly, chest and back.

Continue with your shoulders, arms, throat and neck, face and head.

If you are still feeling tense somewhere in your body, relax and let this tension   go away in the ground.

After relaxing your muscles, feel your body more deeply and allow the internal organs of your abdomen, chest and head to relax.

Listen to your heart and feel its beat becoming slower and more regular, as does your breathing.

Now listen to your breathing and sense the light movements in your body.

Your mind is resting, too.

Supine Positions

Passively accept, as if you were an outsider, any thoughts, images and emotions that may come, letting everything flow, without focussing your attention on anything.

Rest in this position for as long as necessary (quite a few minutes) - mind you stay awake and don't fall asleep.

Now bring your attention back to your breathing, then to the each part of your body, now fully relaxed. Gradually and slowly start moving your feet and hands and then stretch as if you were a cat.

Complete the pose by opening your eyes, then turn on your side and finally sit up.

Experience the feelings of being relaxed.

Benefits: the Savasana pose prepares the mind and the body for the next poses.

The constant practice of the Savasana will bring about a slowing of the heart beat and respiratory rate, the blood pressure will be more balanced. It will allow the the body and both rotator cuffs to be totally relaxed

Jathara Sapivritti Asana or Belly Twist Pose

The supine twist is a variation of the more traditional pose known as 'parivartanasana'

जठरा Abdomen आसन Asana वळण Twist

The Sanskrit word 'Parivartana', which is pronounced pah-ree-Vahr-Tah-nah, means 'Twist'.

From the Savasana pose, bend your knees and bring your heels close to your bottom while keeping your feet on the floor and as wide apart as your hips. Open your arms keeping them on the same line as your shoulders, with your palms facing downwards.

Breathe in, then out, while turning your legs to your right and , after rotating your head to your left, completely relax your knees.

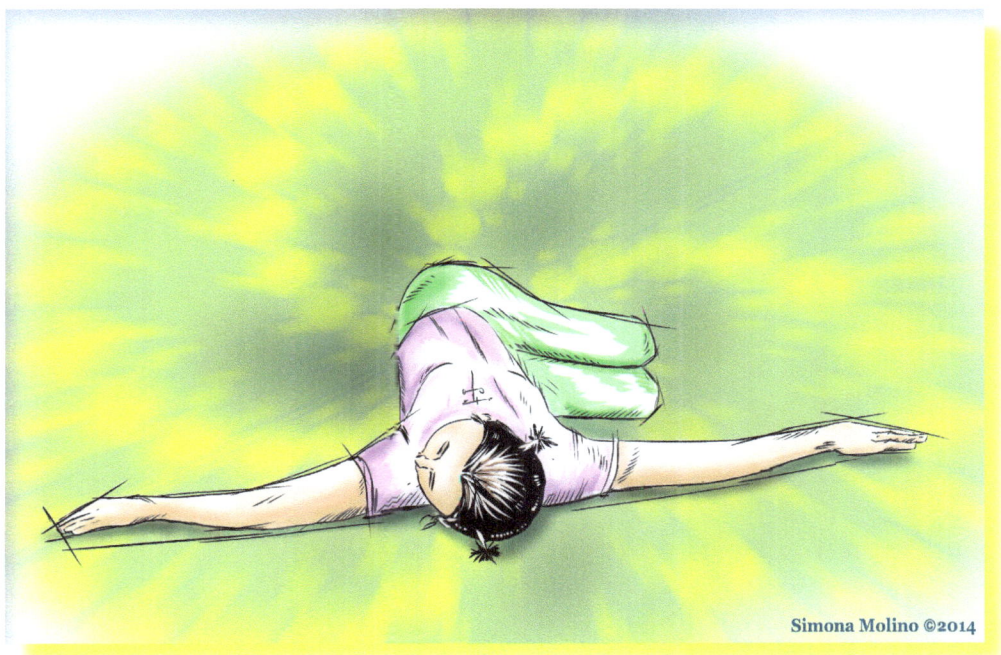

Simona Molino ©2014

Breathe in again, bringing your head and knees back in line.
Breathe out, lowering your legs on the left and turning your head to the right. Repeat the pose for five times, synchronizing the movement of legs and head with your breathing. Relax and return to the initial position.

Benefits: the Belly Twist Movement stretches all your back muscles, re-aligns and extends the spine and hydrates the spinal discs.

Supine Positions

Pavana-mukta-asana or Wind-relieving Pose

The term Pavana-mukta-asana

पवनमुक्तासनम्

freely translated means 'Wind-relieving Pose'
Starting from the previous Savasana pose, close your legs. Breathe in, lifting your right leg and pull it towards your belly slowly and consistently. The left leg stays on the ground.
Pull your right leg from just under your knee with your forearms so

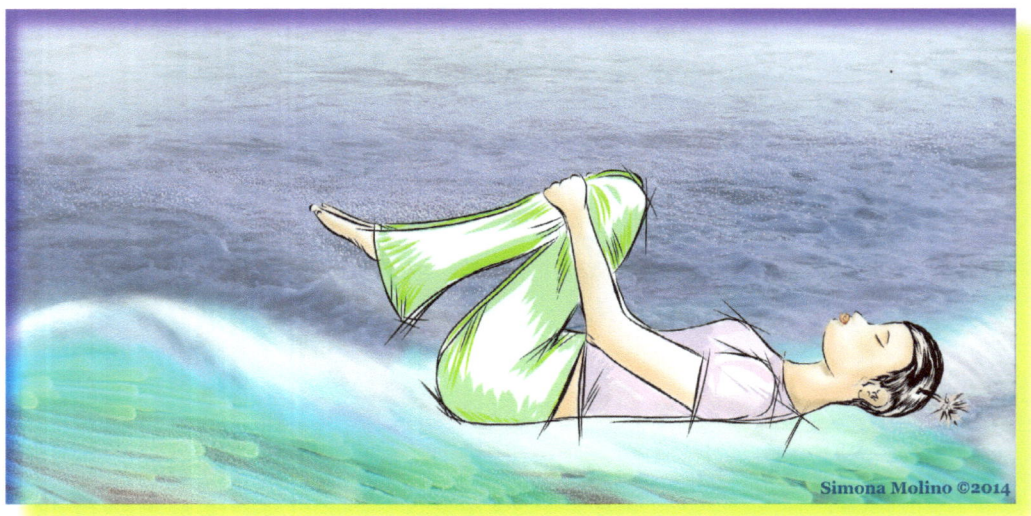

Simona Molino ©2014

that the knee presses against your chest: this gently massages your colon.
Keep your neck and shoulders firmly on the ground.
Keep this position for 1 to 3 breaths.
Breathing out, unlock the position and move your leg slowly back on the ground.
Breathe normally and lie down .
Repeat with your left leg and then with your right leg again and again- three times for each leg.

A possible change to the "Apasana" pose is as follows:

from the "Savasana" pose, close your legs and lift them up by hugging them just above your shins while breathing out.
Keep this position for at least one minute, paying attention to your back, which must be stretched and flat on the ground.
If you feel like it, you may roll backwards and forwards or sideways and give your spine a delicate massage.
Finally, breathe out and release your legs to the ground, then rest.
Repeat up to six times.

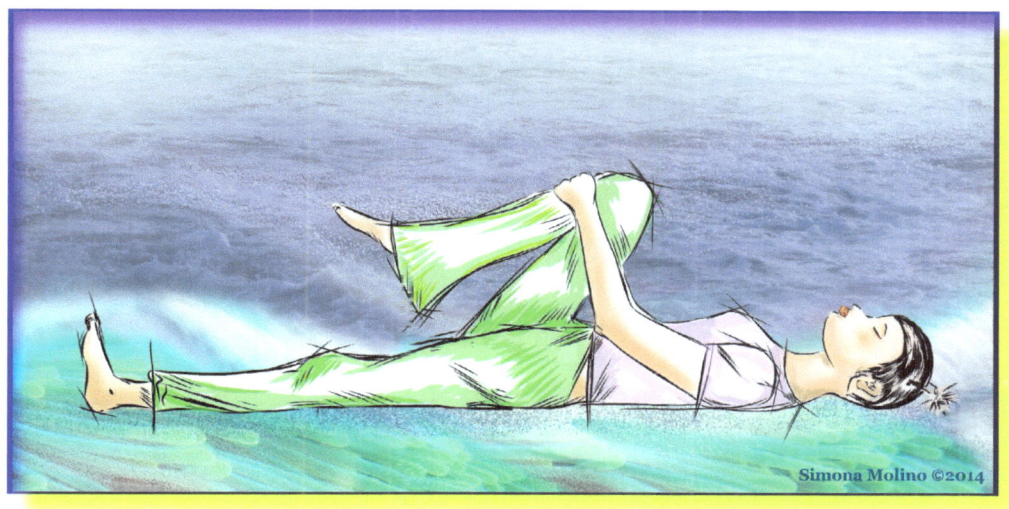

Simona Molino ©2014

Benefits: Practicing this Asana will relax your lower back muscles, your lumbar region, your neck and thigh muscles: it will be just what you need after a long day at a desk and is recommended both before going to bed and as you wake up to encourage your body, mind and spirit to remain pure and balanced all day.

Warning: Do not attempt this position if you have had surgery in your abdomen or a slipped disc.

Also avoid in case of damage to your spine or knee.

Supine Positions

Dvi Pada Pitham Asana or Little Bridge Pose

The name Dvi Pada Pitham Asana comes from Sanskrit and means " position of the Table with Two Legs"

डीवीआईप्रदर्शक

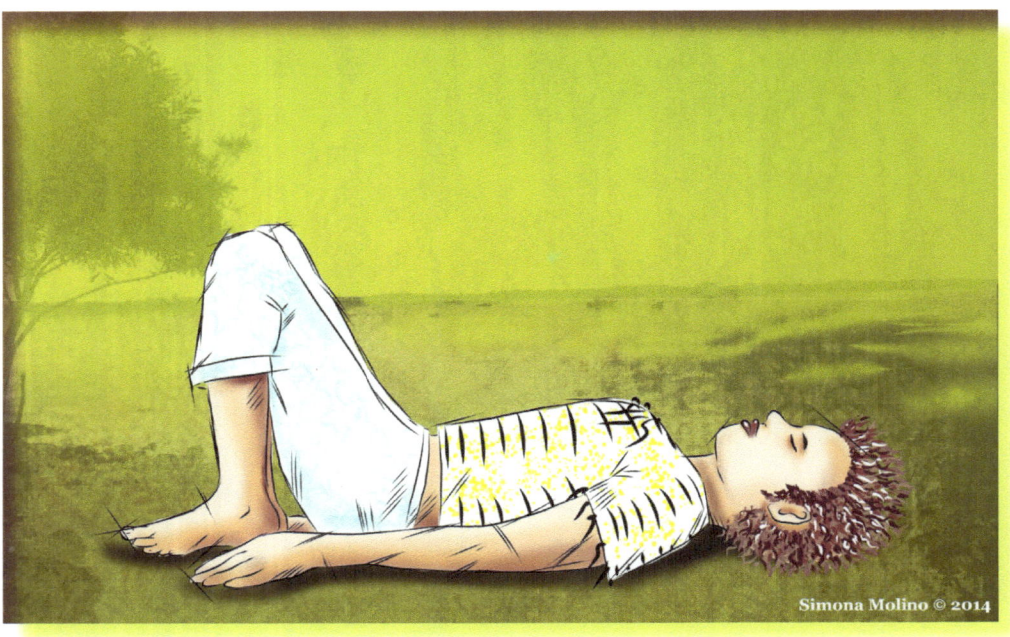

Simona Molino © 2014

From the Savanasana or Apasana Pose, bend your knees with your legs as far apart as your hips and place them perpendicular to your heels. Thighs and bottom are parallel.
Lower your chin towards your throat without raising your head.
Breathe in and out, concentrating on your breathing.
While breathing out, put pressure on your soles so that your lumbar curve adheres to the ground. Breathing in, raise your pelvis, then your lumbar curve and part of your back keeping your legs parallel.

Keep this static position for a few breaths, then breathe out and put your bottom on the ground.
Repeat five times.
Relax in the Savasana Pose.

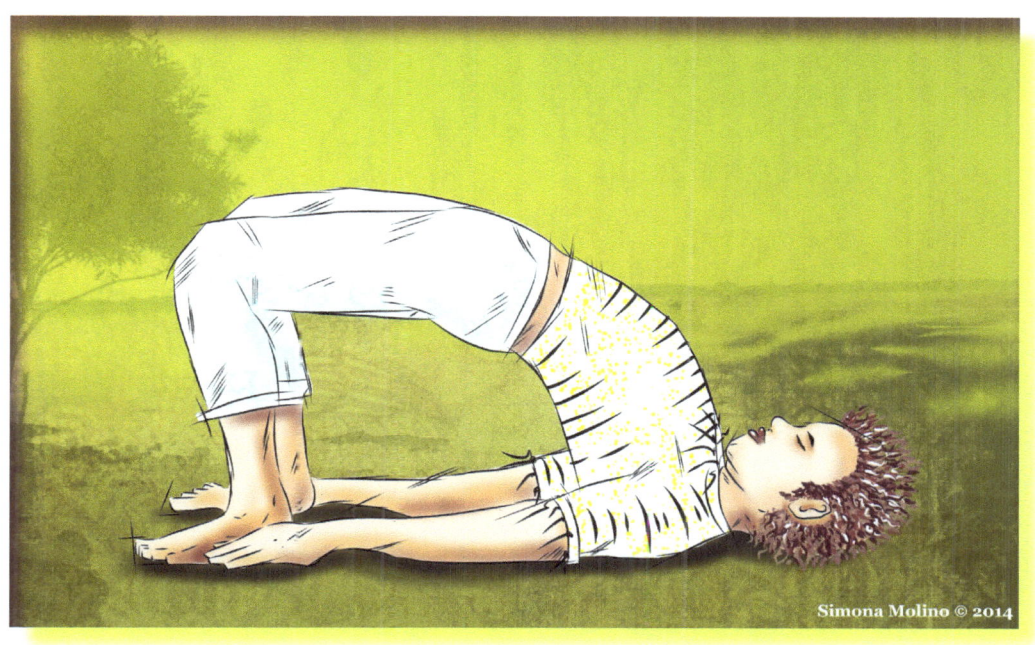

Simona Molino © 2014

Benefits: Dvi Pada Pitham Asana expands your chest, neck and spine; reduces backache and stress in general.

Warning: Do not attempt if you have known neck lesions - only assume this position under the direct supervision of an expert teacher.

Supine Positions

Adavasana or Reverse Corpse Pose

The Sanskrit word "Adava Asaba" means "Prone or reverse Pose"

अद्वासन Prone Pose

Like Savasana, this pose is meant to relax both body and mind.
Lie down prone: my advice is to use two rolled up towels in a V form
to position your face and allow you to breathe freely.
The neck must be relaxed.
Arms and hands can be put at the sides with palms up - or loosely
stretched above your head if you feel more comfortable.

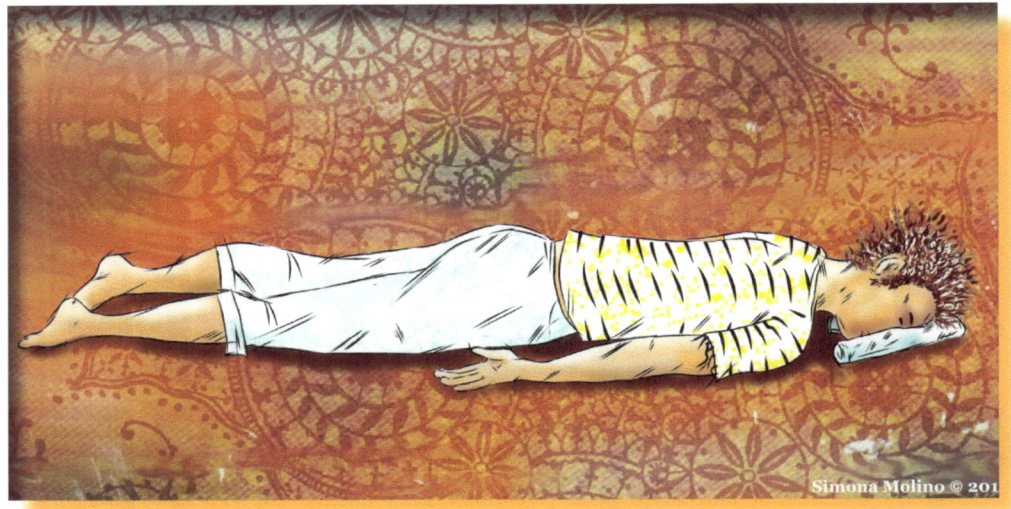

Relax and abandon yourself like in Savasana.
Your stomach touches the ground lightly.
Breathe deeply and feel your belly press against the ground when
you breathe in - let the muscles of your lower back, legs and face relax
completely.
Keep this position for three minutes at least.
To release the position, put your hands at the sides and slowly rise
bending your knees and sitting on your heels.

Benefits: This pose is beneficial if you suffer from a slipped disc, neck tensions and if you stay all day in a curved posture.

Warning: Be cautious if you suffer from stenosis, as this position can worsen nerve compression.

Naga-Asana or Cobra or Snake Pose

The Sanskrit word naga means snake or serpent.

Naga-asana is also known as Bhujanga-asana. The Sanskrit word Bhujanga, which also means snake, is derived from the root bhuj, which means to bend or curve.

Bhujanga Snake साप Asana आसन

At first, keep your arms alongside the body with palms facing down and lift your head and chest off the ground.

Bend your arms and put your hands at the side of your head and your

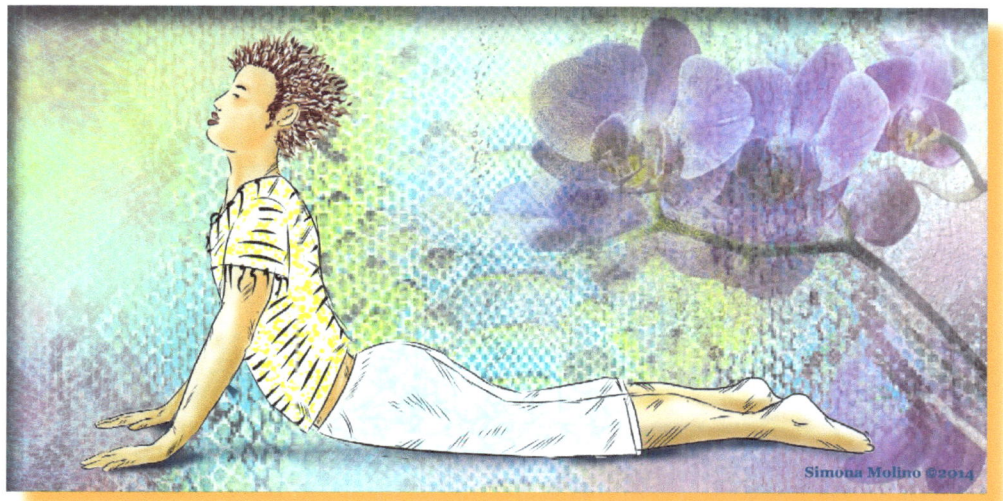

Simona Molino ©2014

elbows at the side of your trunk.

Breathe in and press down on your palms lifting your head and chest off the ground, your shoulders are lowered and the pubic bone touches the ground. Your chest is slightly thrust forward.

Look up. Relax shoulders and legs. Keep this position listening to your breathing for at least 10 breathing cycles. Breathe out and release the pose by putting back your belly, shoulders chin and forehead on the ground.

Benefits: The Cobra or Snake pose is beneficial to the spine, tones up the lower back and lumbar muscles. If you are diabetic, you will find this pose greatly helps you stimulate blood circulation in your gonad, adrenal, thyroid glands and pancreas.

Warning: Do not attempt if you have had recent fractures or knee, shoulder or arm problems and if you have undergone abdominal surgery. This pose is also not advised if you suffer from hyperthyroidism, peptic ulcer and hernia, carpal tunnel syndrome and headache and if you are pregnant.

Prone Positions

Dandasana or Staff Pose

The name "dandasana" comes from the Sanskrit, from the terms "danda" means "Staff" and "Asana" pose.

दन्द Staff आसन Asana

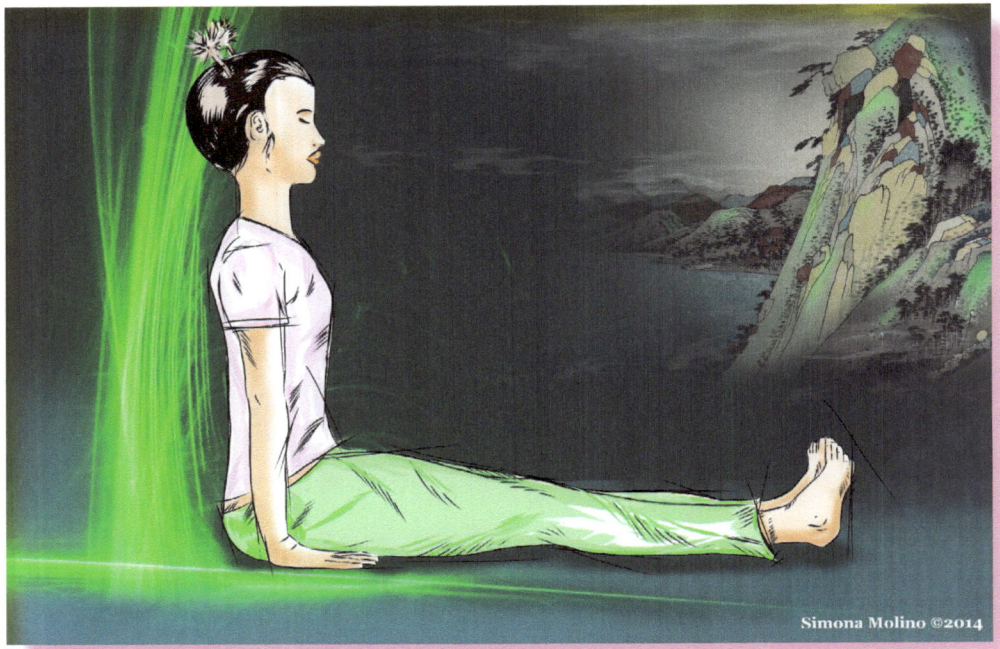

Simona Molino ©2014

Sit with your legs closed and stretched in front of you, toes upwards and feet at a 90 degree angle with the ground. Arms along your sides and hands with palms on the ground or on your knees.

Stretch your back upwards with relaxed shoulders, with your chin parallel to the ground so that both nape and tailbone are aligned. You may find it helpful, especially at first, to sit with your back leaning onto a wall. Always make sure that tailbone and shoulder blades touch the wall.

Balance your body weight on both hips and feel the hip bone pressed on the ground. Keep this position concentrating on your breathing. Breathe in and feel your spine elongating upwards, your chest lifts up as it expands. Breathe out and feel your belly empty while contracting towards your spine.

Benefits: Dandasana will help your posture, strengthen your back muscles, favour digestion, prevent sciatic pain; it will elongate and activate your leg muscles and prevent tired feet and shin muscles.

Warning: Do not attempt if you have lower back pains.

Pascimottanasana or Caterpillar Pose

The name Pascimottanâsana derives from the Sanskrit

पश्चिम That which is in the West उत्तान Open, Stretched आसन Asana

Starting from the Dandasana pose, breathe in and lift up your arms towards the Sky, stretching your spine upwards.

Breathing out, slowly bend your bust, including your hips. Stretch your coccyx distancing it from the back of your pelvis. Your hands reach out for your toes: if you can, grab the outside of your feet. If you can't, place your hands on your thighs, calves or ankles, depending on your flexibility.

Maintain this static position, breathing normally.

Breathe in, then slowly and gradually return to the initial position.

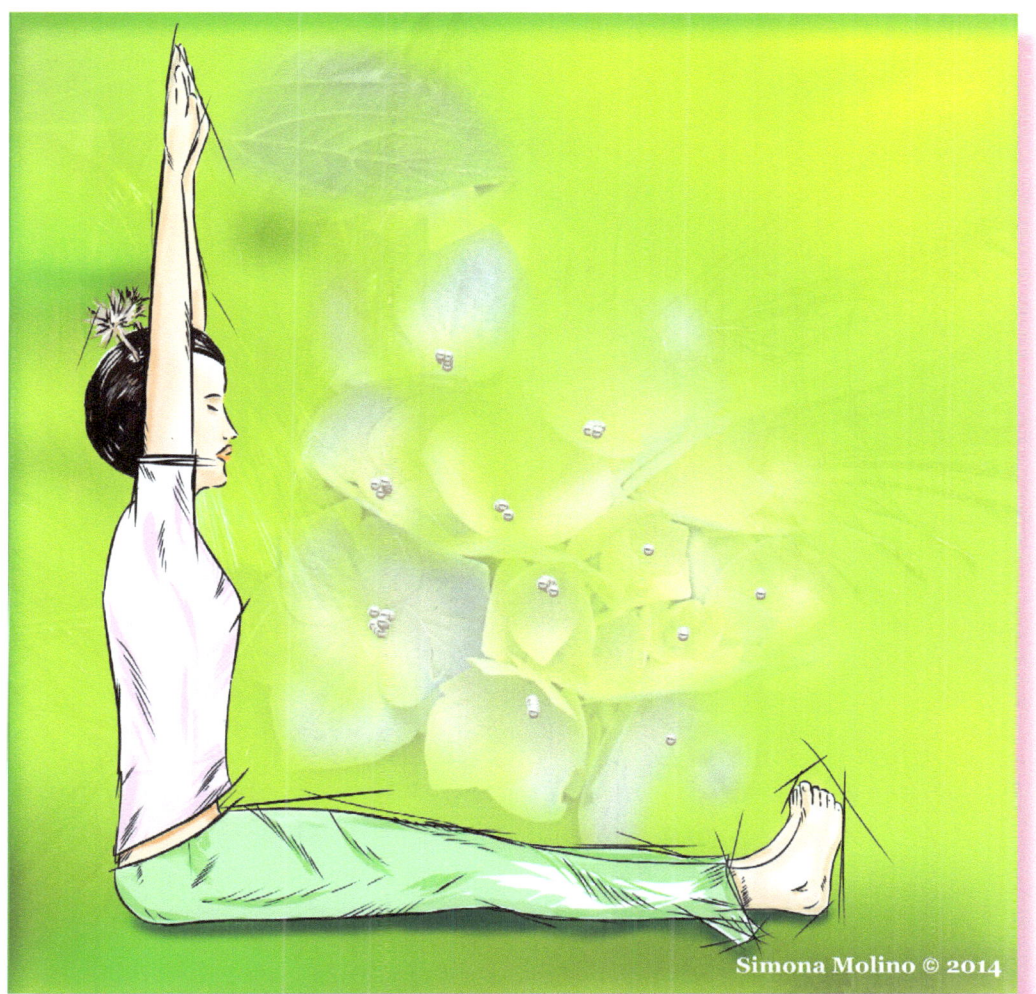

Simona Molino © 2014

Sitting Positions

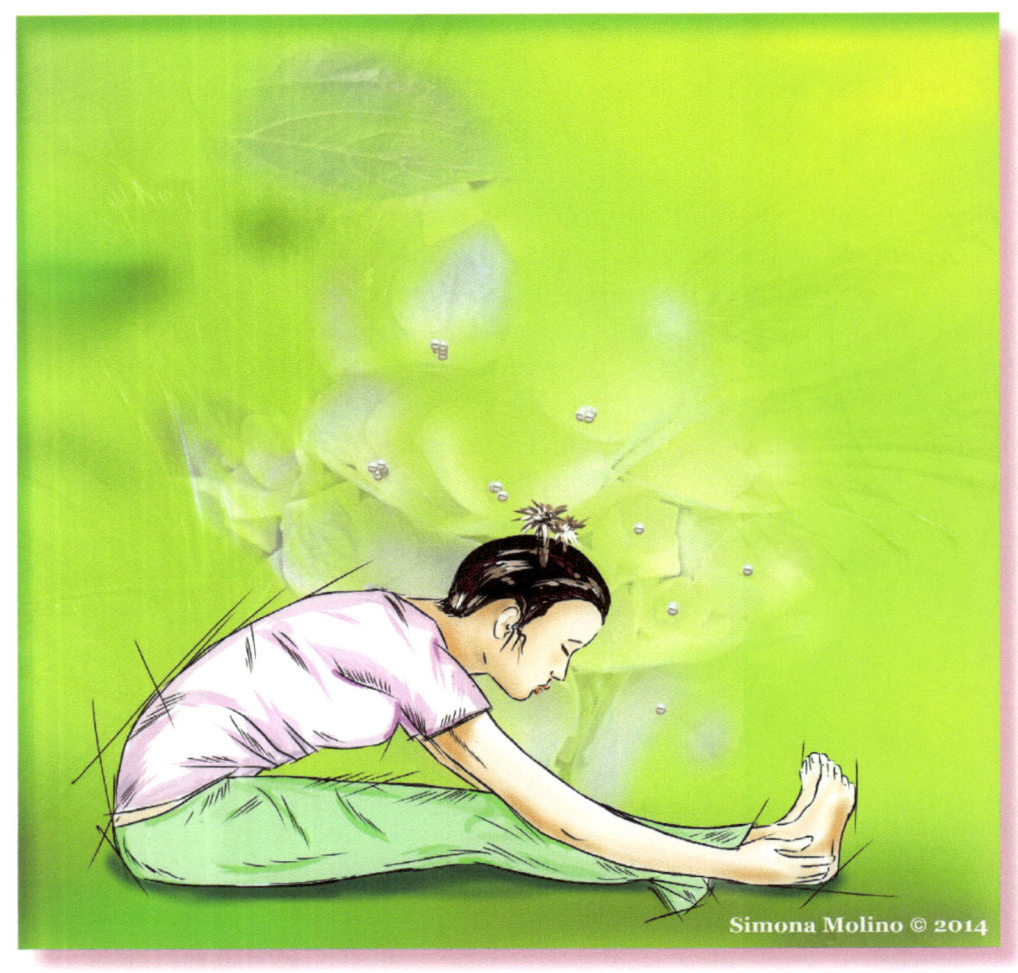

Simona Molino © 2014

Benefits: Pascimottanasana has positive effects on your prostate, releases your sciatic nerve, stretches out lordosis, helps to control anxiety, stretches the leg and back muscles and tendons and promotes fact reduction round your belly and hips.

Warning: Avoid this pose if suffering from slipped disc.

Tadasana or Mountain Pose

The name Tadasana derives from the Sanskrit

पर्वताची रांग **Mountain** आसन **Asana**

'Tada' means 'Mountain' and 'Asana' 'Position'; this asana is also known as samasthitiâsana, where 'Sama' means 'Static' or 'Balance' and 'Sthiti' means the Act of standing firmly still.

Tadasana, or Mountain pose, represents our basic standing posture. Stand up with legs closed and toes almost touching each other. Now put your feet as wide apart as to be in line with your shoulders, always keeping them parallel to each other.

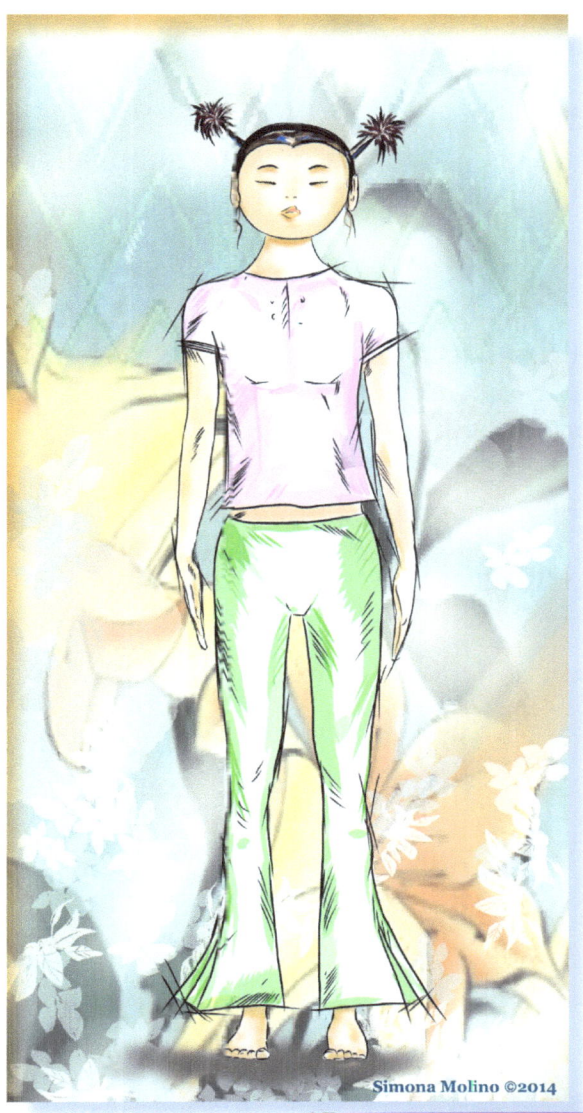

Simona Molino ©2014

17

Standing Positions

Legs and knees are relaxed.

Slightly move your arms away from your trunk and close your eyes, focussing on your feet. Lift your toes, stretch them and then gently put them back on the ground.

Feel your body weight drop by extending your coccyx downwards. The pelvis lifts towards the navel.

Widen your collarbones and let them slide down, towards your back. Head and bust are aligned, the head is above the centre of the pelvis. The throat is de-stressed and the tongue relaxed and flat on the bottom of the mouth.

Move the weight of your body forwards and backwards, then to the right and the left and feel how it balances on your feet and which muscles are tense or contracted.

Keep moving with a concentric circular movement until you reach the Centre.

Close you eyes and let them relax.

Keep this position for a few minutes, breathing normally.

Benefits: Tadasana develops physical and emotional balance, strengthens thighs, knees and ankles, tones up abdominal and gluteus muscles, alleviates sciatic nerve pains.

Warning: Don't perform with headache, sleeplessness or low blood pressure.

KalaAsana or Time Pose

The name Kala asana derives from the Sanskrit

वेळ Time आसन asana

'Kala' means 'Time'.
Standing up, start with the Tadasana pose.
Close your eyes. Breathe in and bring your weight onto your right foot,

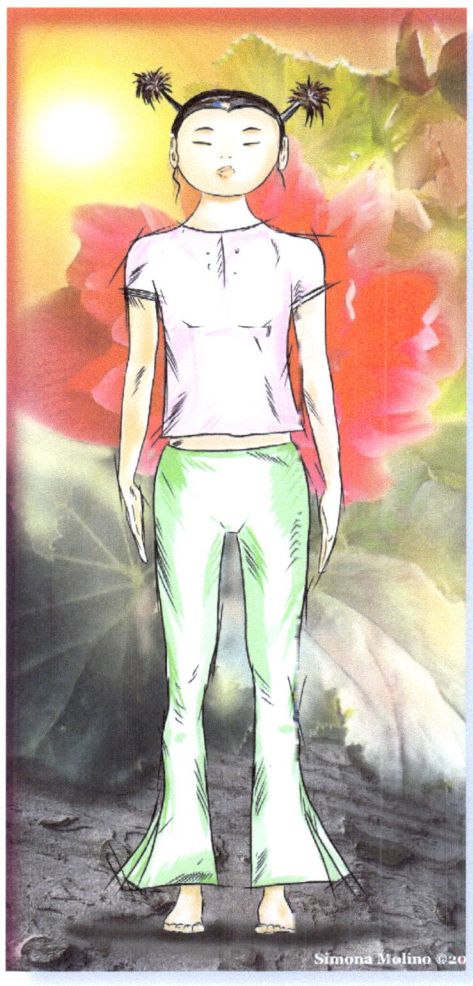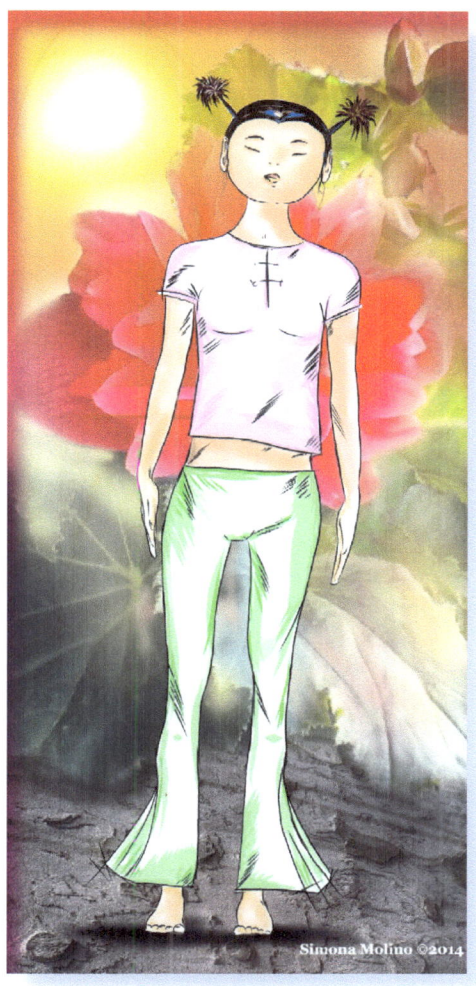

breathe out and feel how light the left side of your body becomes ; then again breathe in and bring the weight onto your left foot, breathe out noticing the lightness of you right side.
Repeat five times.

Benefits: helps fight sleeplessness and strengthens balance.

Standing Positions

Padahastana or Hand Under Foot Pose

The meaning of the word Padahastasana comes from the Sanskrit 'Pada', meaning Feet, and 'Hasta', meaning Hands.

पाद Feet हस्ता Hands

In the Tadasana pose, breathe in and stretch your arms above your head keeping them next to your ears and with palms facing front. Breathe out and bend over towards Earth with your head, neck and

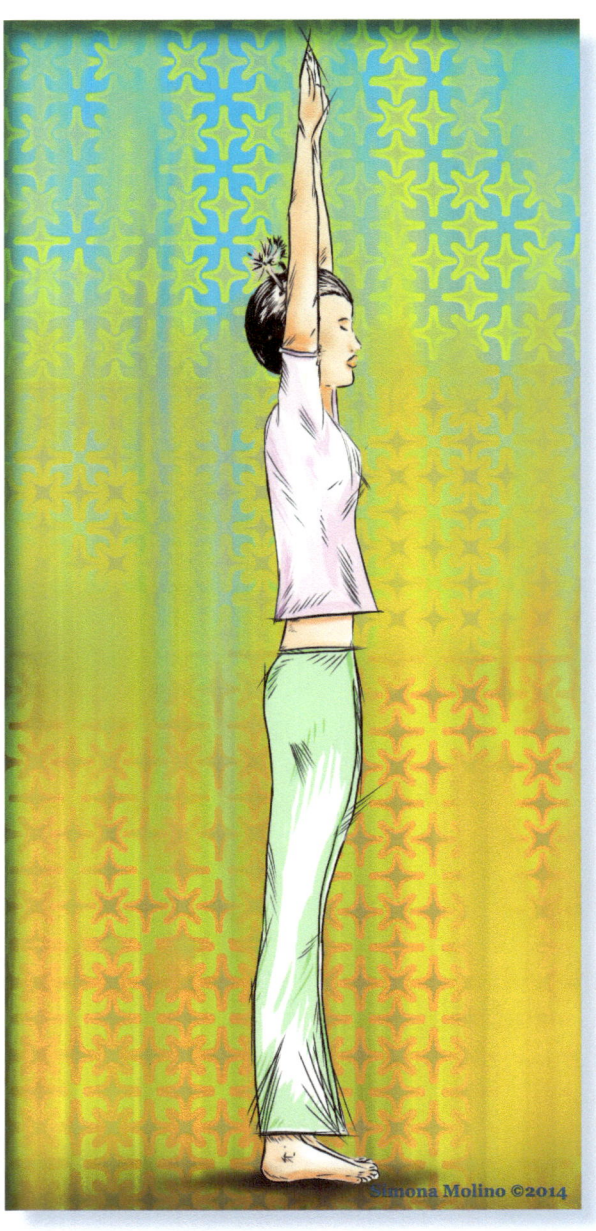

spine, until your palms or fingers touch the ground next to the side of your feet.

Keep your legs straight, slightly drawing your knees in.

Maintain this position for a few seconds.

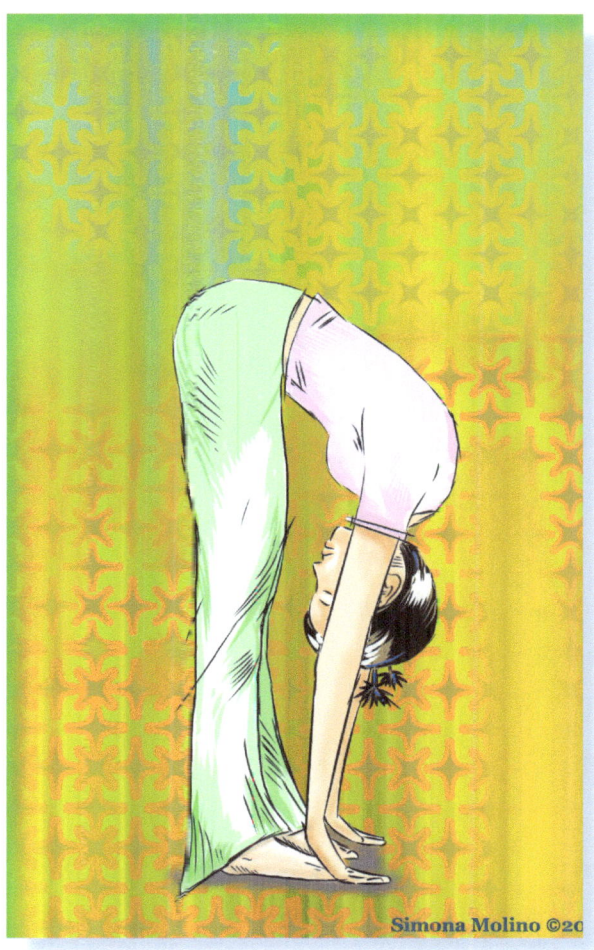

Benefits: it alleviates back pains, stretches the spine, betters nerve pain. Padasthasana also improves bloodflow and facilitates the oxygenation of head and face. It also stretches leg muscles and tendons and increases spine elasticity and flexibility. All the organs in the abdomen, such as intestine and stomach, are stimulated and toned, digestive and intestinal functions greatly improve.

Warning: People suffering from serious back conditions (hernia) should not bend over completely. They can bend over from the hips, while keeping the back straight, creating a 90-degree angle with the legs. Padasthasana is unsafe if you are suffering from low blood pressure.

Standing Positions

Namaskarasana or Prayer Squat Pose

Namaskarasana or Prayer Squat Pose

आसन Asana नमस्कार Greeting

From the Tadasana Pose, place your feet at a 45-degree angle and as wide apart as your shoulders. Kneel, keeping your elbows inside your kees.

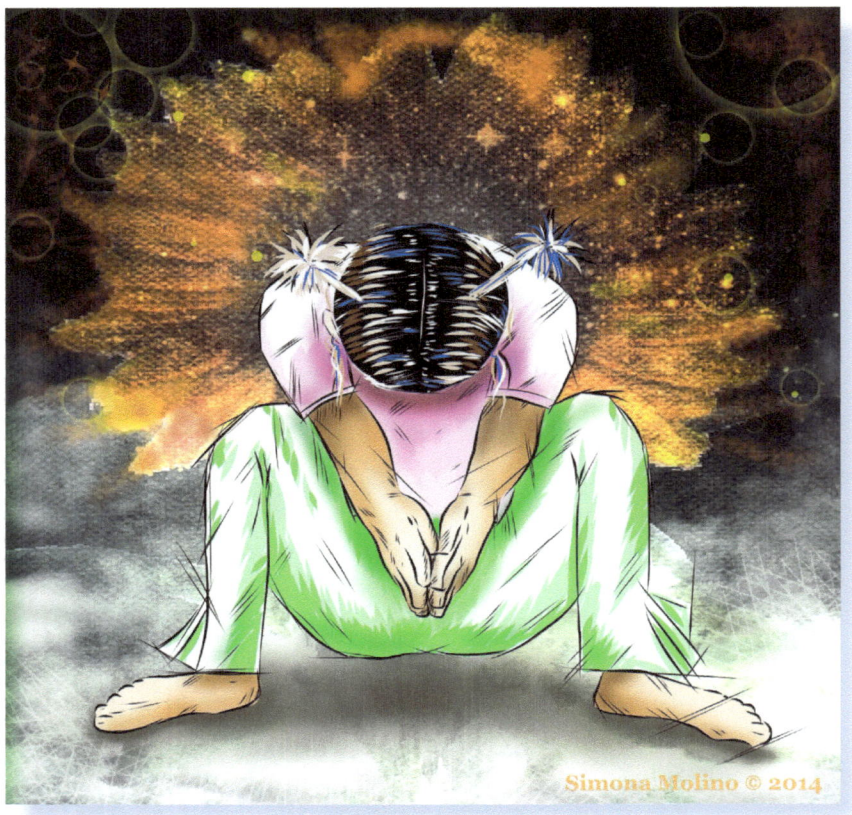

Put your hands before your chest, with your head slightly tilted backwards, feeling the pressure of your elbows on your knees.
Breathe out and straighten your arms in front of you, then bend your head and press it on your chest.
Keep this pose for a few breaths, feeling your shoulder and top of your back muscles.
Breathe in and slowly return to the Tadasana Pose.
Repeat at least five times.

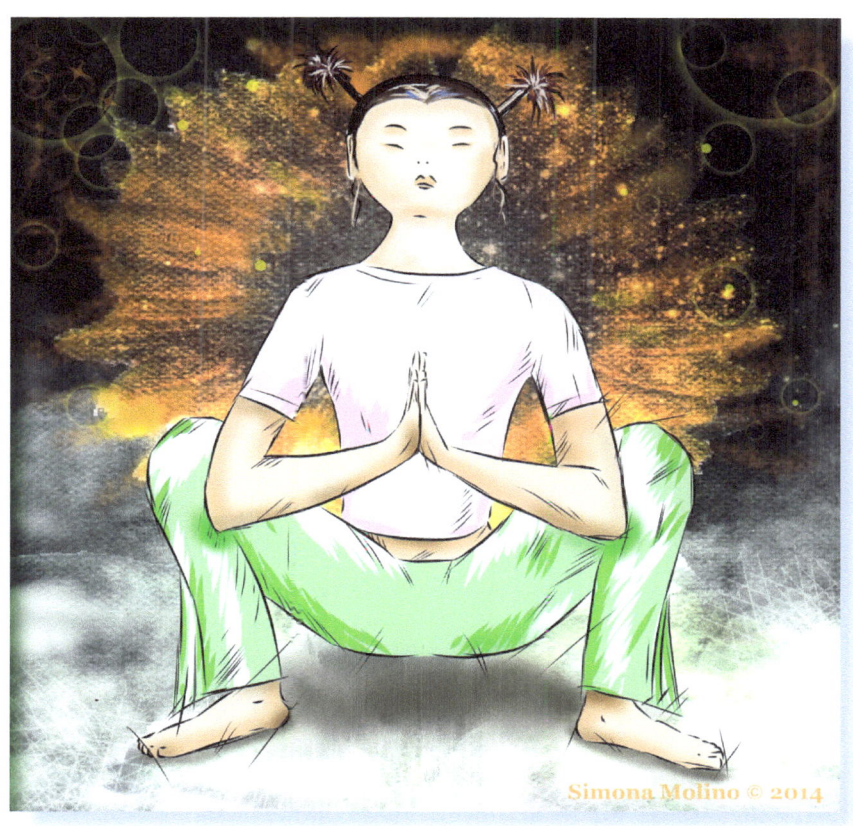

Simona Molino © 2014

Benefits: Namaskarasana calms your nerves and tones your thigh, knee, shoulder, arm and neck muscles. It enhances hips flexibility.

Warning: Do not attempt if you suffer from sciatica pain or have known knee problems.

Standing Positions

Balasana or Child's Pose

The word 'bala asana' originates from Sanskrit and means 'Child's Pose'.

बालासन Child's pose

Sit on your heels with your legs closed, feet stretched backwards and

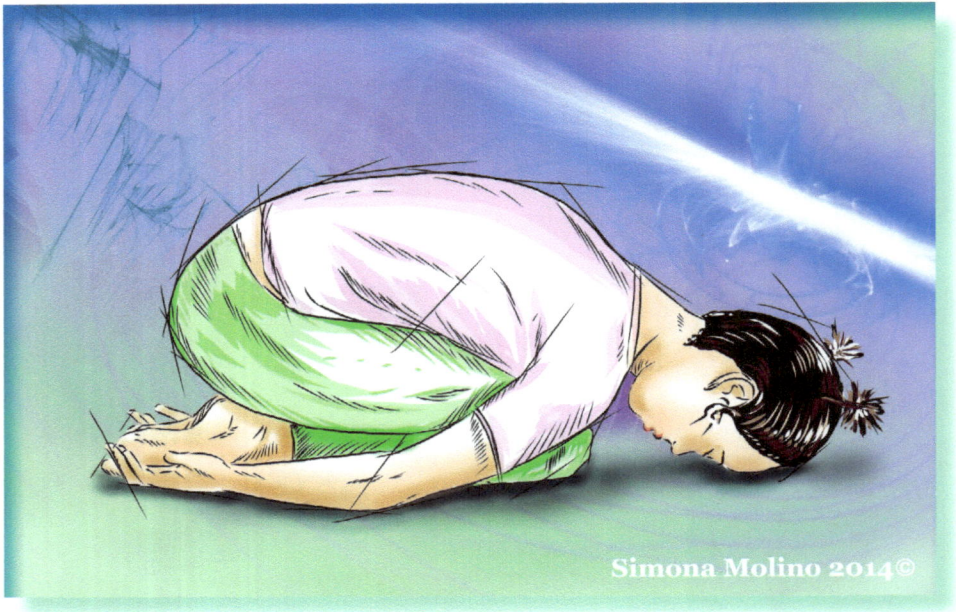

Simona Molino 2014©

slightly apart, big toes touching. Now widen your knees in line with your hips. The gluteus muscles sit on the hollow of your heels.

Breathe out and gently bend over until you touch the floor close to your knees with your forehead. Stretch your arms back, close to your body, with your palms facing downwards.

Keep this static position for about thirty seconds, breathing normally. Relax and let yourself go.

Slowly return to the sitting position and, starting from the bottom, loosen one vertebra after the other leaving the head to come up last.

A tip: if you find it too difficult to reach the ground with your forehead, you can put a blanket or some cushions under your bottom.

Benefits: This pose leads to a passive lengthening of the paraspinal muscles, found at the sides of the spine, which can often feel tense after an active day. All muscles in the back will benefit, the spine will be loosened as the pose creates a wider space between the intervertebral discs and helps fight their physiological deterioration.

Warning: Don't attempt to do this if you have a slipped disc, spondylosis or spondylolisthesis.

Shashankasana or Hare Pose

The name Shashankasana comes from the Sanskrit

शशांकासन

and means "position that frees from the air"

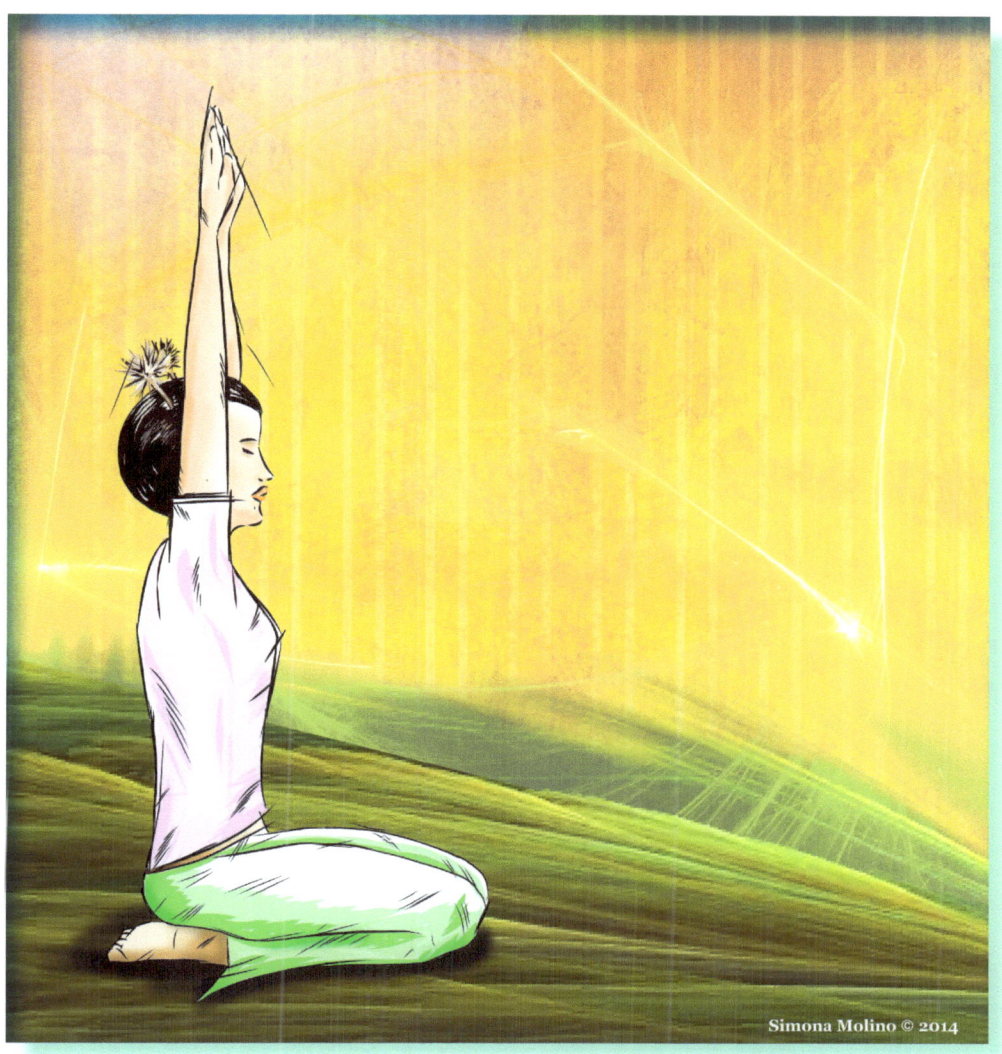

Simona Molino © 2014

Kneel down and put your hands on your knees.
Breathe in and raise your hands vertically above your head. Breathe out while bending your trunk forwards, keeping your arms in line with your trunk.
Your forehead touches the ground, arms and hands relax at the side of your head with palms facing downwards.

25

Kneeling Positions

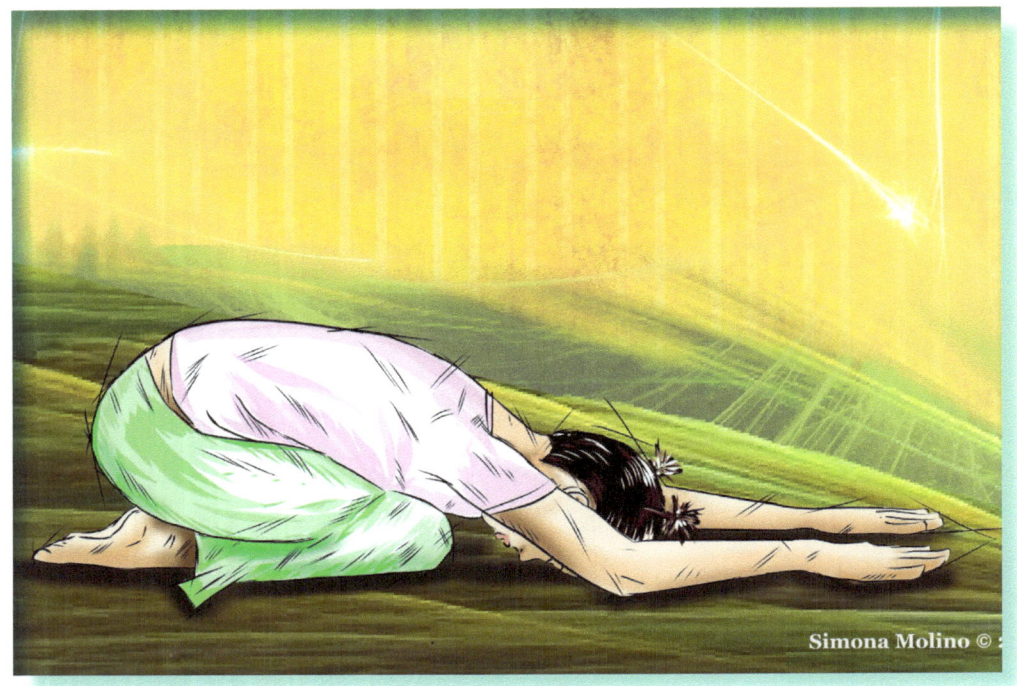

Simona Molino ©

Maintain this pose, relaxing shoulders, back, neck, head and arms for a few breaths.
Slowly breathe out and go back to your initial pose, lowering your arms.
Repeat this asana up to ten times.

Benefits: this asana helps relax your back muscles; it also alleviates tiredness and favours concentration.

Warning: Do not attempt if you have high blood pressure, glaucoma or vertigo.

Bidalasana or Cat Pose

The name Bidalasana comes from the Sanskrit words

बिडाल Cat आसन Asana

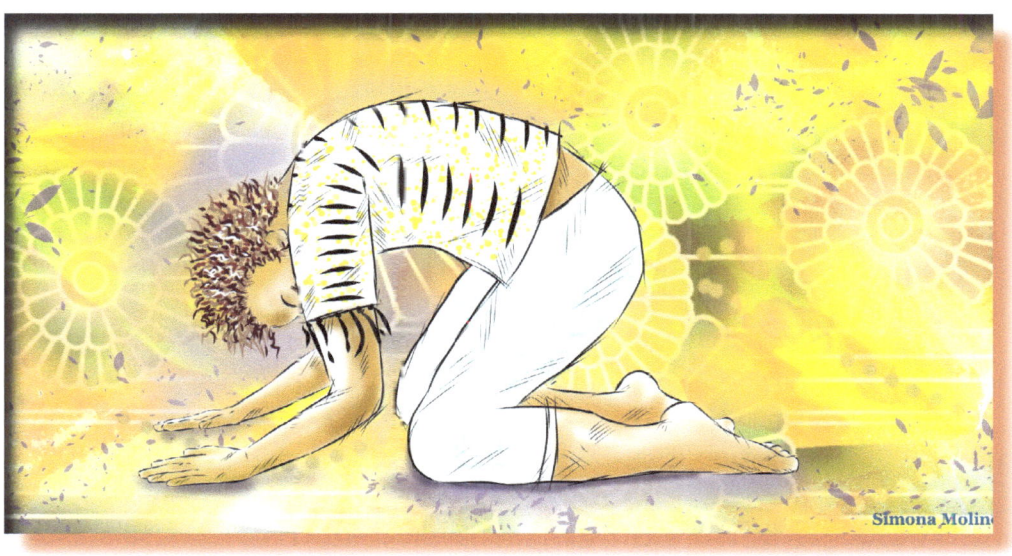

Simona Molin

Assume the kneeling position with your hands on the ground and your back curved.

Make sure your hips are behind your knees, as to feel a very light weight on your hands.

Your arms must be relaxed, starting from your shoulders, to your elbows and hands.

Inhale and start moving your back from your shoulders, expand your chest, and then gradually and slowly continue moving your back to your hips.

Your back must be uniformly stretched, as if you were trying to separate one vertebra from the other.

Your neck could be lightly stretched and lifted at the end of the movement.

Quadrupedal Positions

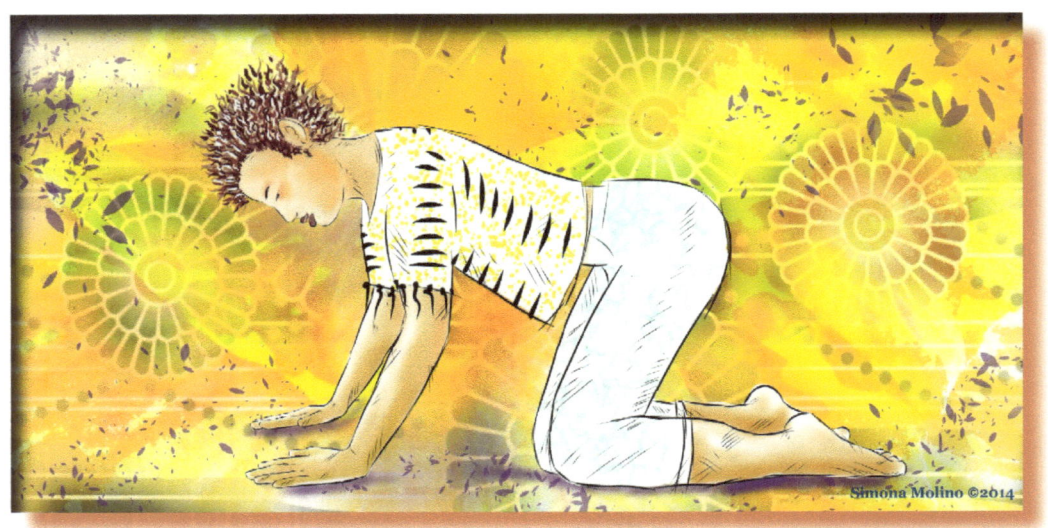

Breathing out, carefully start repeating the sequence in the opposite direction, starting with your hips, sliding backwards, followed by back and shoulders.

Your head should come close to the breastbone.

Repeat the whole pose five times.

When you want to take a break, you can assume the Balasana back rest pose.

Benefits: Bidalasana makes the whole spine more sensitive, increasing its elasticity by compressing and extending its back and front areas. It also makes the chest more elastic by increasing its breathing capacity.

Bidalasana is a safe pose even for pregnant women as it is extremely useful during labour to help the baby in the canal during delivery.

Elongating Pose

Assume this pose if you have been sitting too long in a contracted position or just to relax your body and wake it up again.

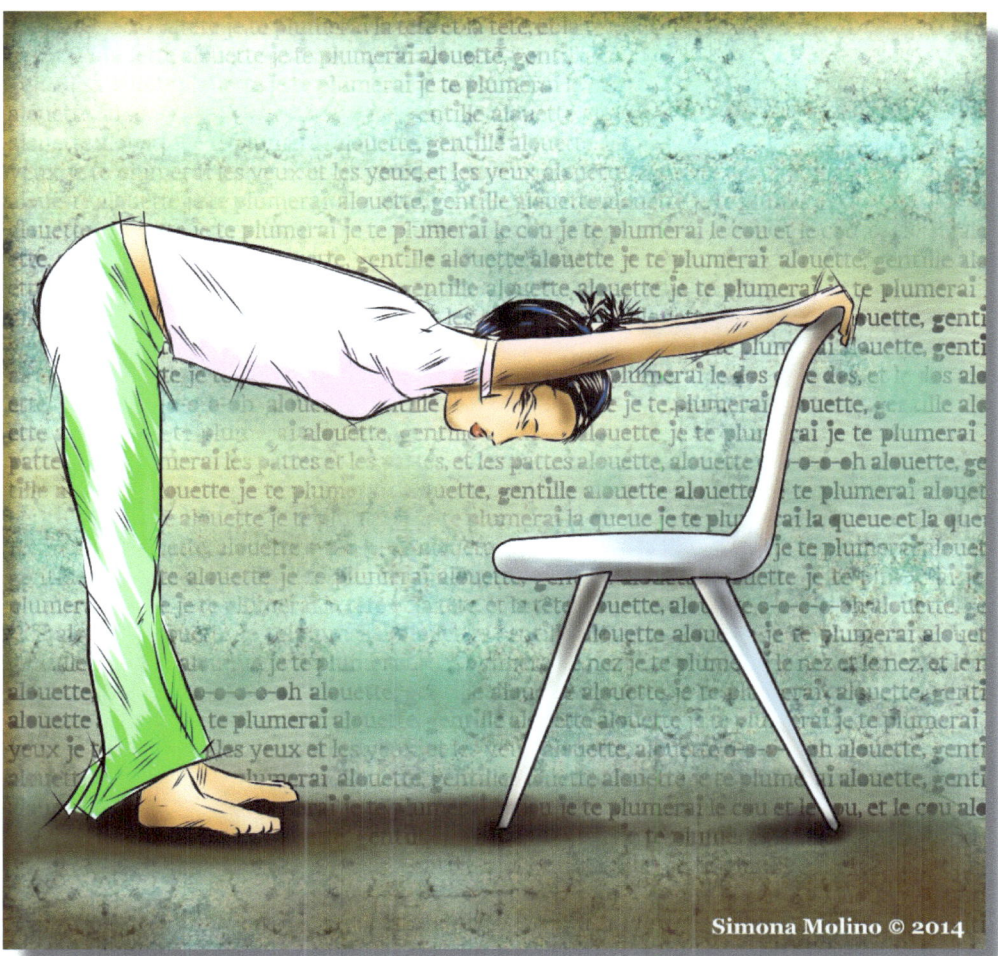

Simona Molino © 2014

Stand in a front of a chair, spread your legs as wide as your hips and put your hands on top of the back of the chair, bend forwards and relax your back.

Feel your back elongate , relax your head. Your trunk is straight and in line with your arms.

Breathe in and out keeping this position for at least 5 to 10 breaths.

Benefits: This pose relaxes your spine and stretches your arms,shoulders and legs, relaxes muscular tensions, and prevents cramps.

Office Pose

Uktanasana or Chair pose

The word Uktanasana comes from the Sanskrit

उत्कट heave o intense आसन Asana

This asana, which may look gentle at first, is actually intense and vibrant.
You can practise a lighter version during the day to ease tension.
This version is as follows:
Standing with your shoulders to a wall, feet and heels touching the
wall, take a little step forward.
Breathe out and bend your knees as to have your thighs parallel to the
wall and your knees perpendicular to your heels.

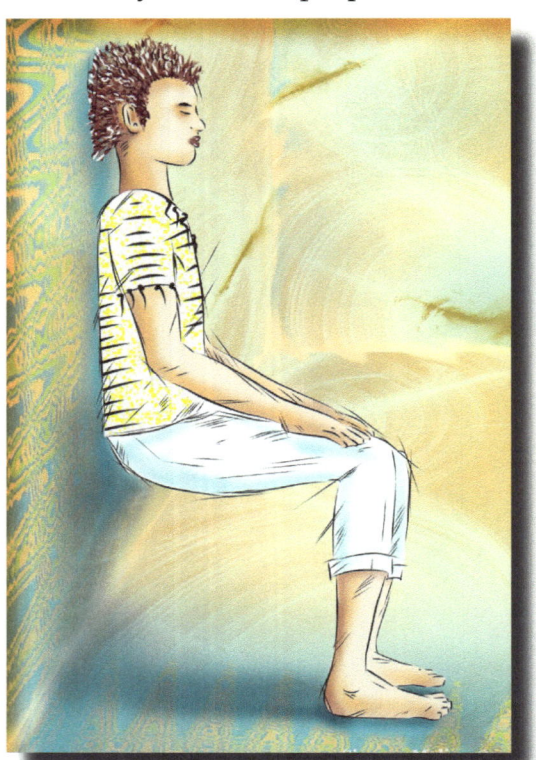 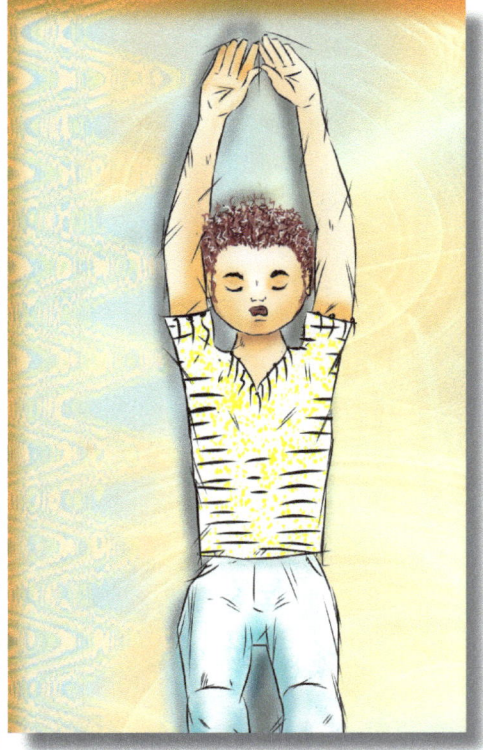

Adhere close to the wall so that your sacral zone touches the wall,
breathe in and raise your arms upwards, keeping your spine to the
wall and your chin slightly down.
Keep this position for 5 to 10 breathing cycles feeling the sensations in
your body.

*Benefits: this position stretches your whole spine , relaxes shoulders,
strengthens legs and lumbar area. Very good to relax if you have been
sitting for a long time or in uncomfortable positions.*

Arm stretching while you are sitting

This practice helps to relax back, arms, shoulders and hands when must sit for a long time or you have to maintain tense or uncomfortable positions.

You can practice this position even while you are sitting down.

I personally do this while I am jogging or running to relax my arms and expand my chest.

Join your hands as if praying and cross your fingers.

Turn your palms upwards and outwards.

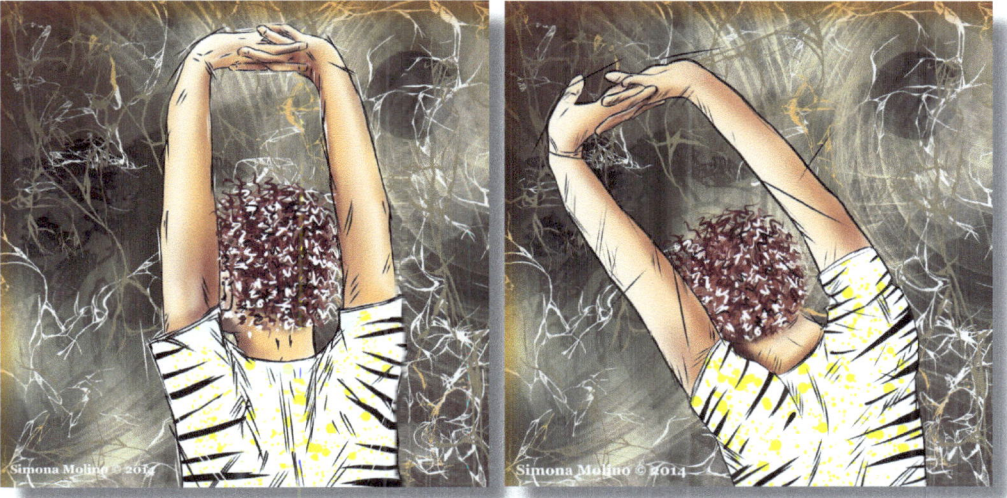

Straighten your arms and hands above your head.

Keep this position and breathe deeply a few times, in and out.

Stretch your right and left sides while keeping your hands above your head.

Breathe in and out while stretching your sides.

Simona Molino

I was born in 1969 - the Year of the Moon -
Since childhood I have always loved drawing animals, especially small horses...now I prefer little frogs!
In 2004 I founded an art studio, Studio Artistico Janas, drawing from the "Janas" or fairy of Sardinian tradition and her magic flight.
I am an Author, Illustrator, Decorator and Graphic Designer, I live and work near Milan with my human and furry family.
My illustrated works in e-book format and paperback are edited on the Amazon platform and they are translated into English, French and German.
For many years now I have been practicing Bio-Disciplines like Tai Chi Chuan, Reiki and Yoga.
How to contact me: janasart@yahoo.it
www.studioartisticojanas.com

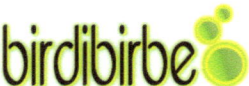

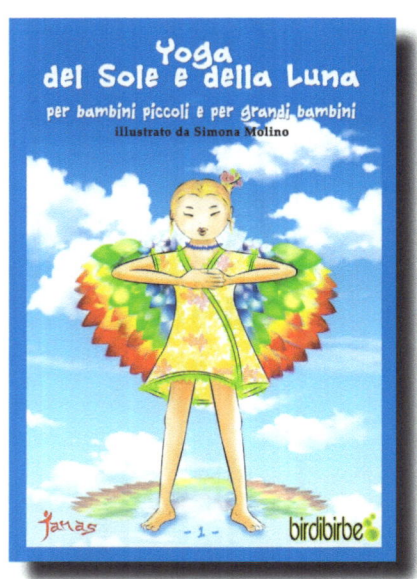

Sun Practices are recommended for children and adults who don't exercise very much, for grumpy children or children who cry too easily, or to start the day creatively and enthusiastically.

The Moon Practices are for the day or the evening, for adults or children who feel stressed or need to channel their energy and find a balance between affectivity and receptivity.

If you practice at night, they will ease you into a sweet sleep and deep rest.

A handbook to practice yoga for the little ones and not so little ones anymore, who want to treat themselves to a space where they can relax body and mind.

The texts guide the reader step by step and and explain very clearly how to preform The Sun and Moon Practices, the colourful illustrations attract children's interest and attention.

Suitable from three years of age.

available in ebook and paperback

www.ingramcontent.com/pod-product-compliance
Lightning Source LLC
Chambersburg PA
CBHW060805290526
45792CB00005BA/1527